This is your BODY.

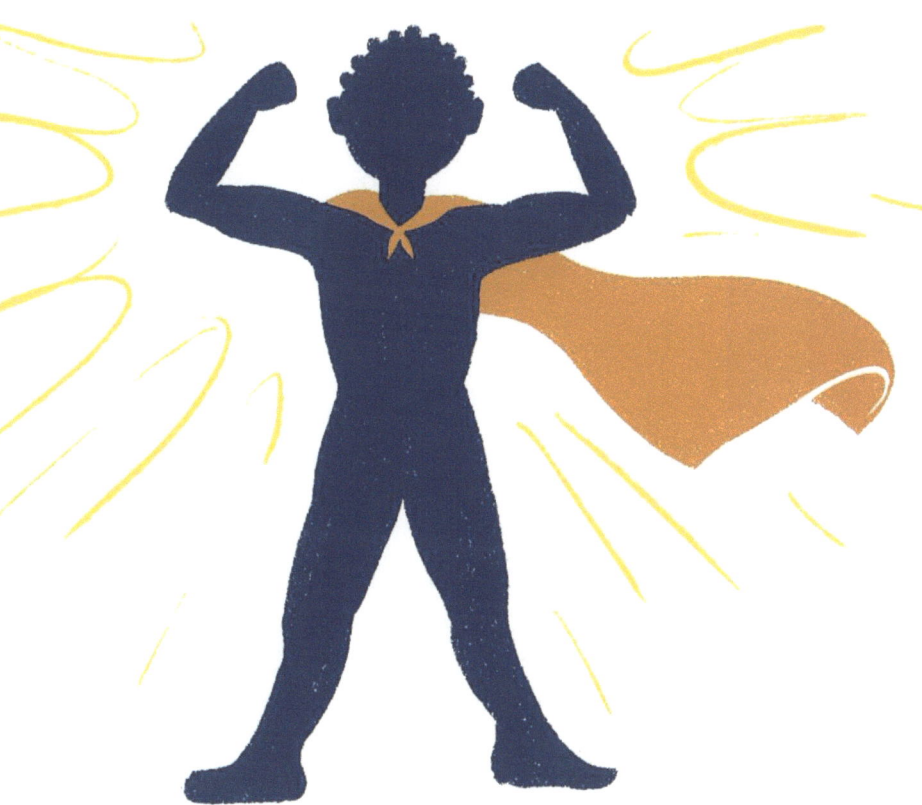

YOUR **BODY** IS MADE UP OF BONES,

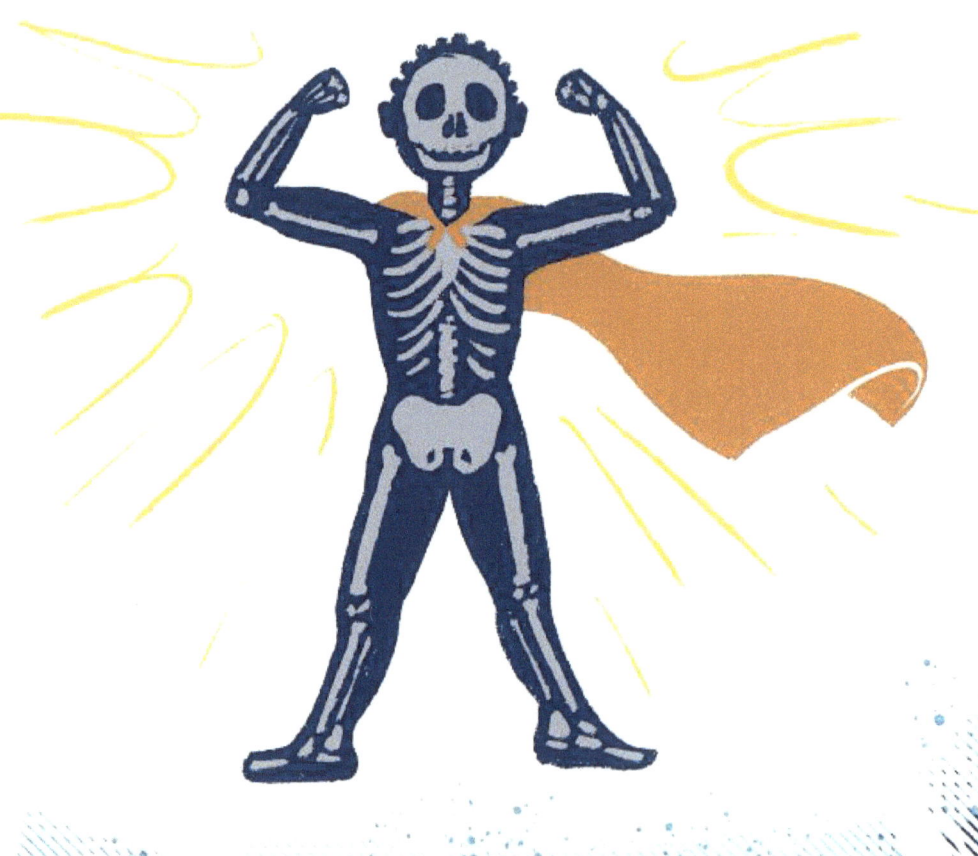

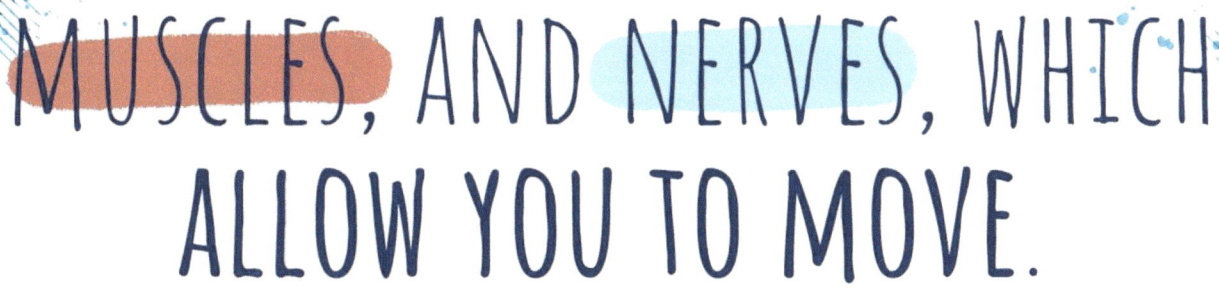

MUSCLES, AND NERVES, WHICH ALLOW YOU TO MOVE.

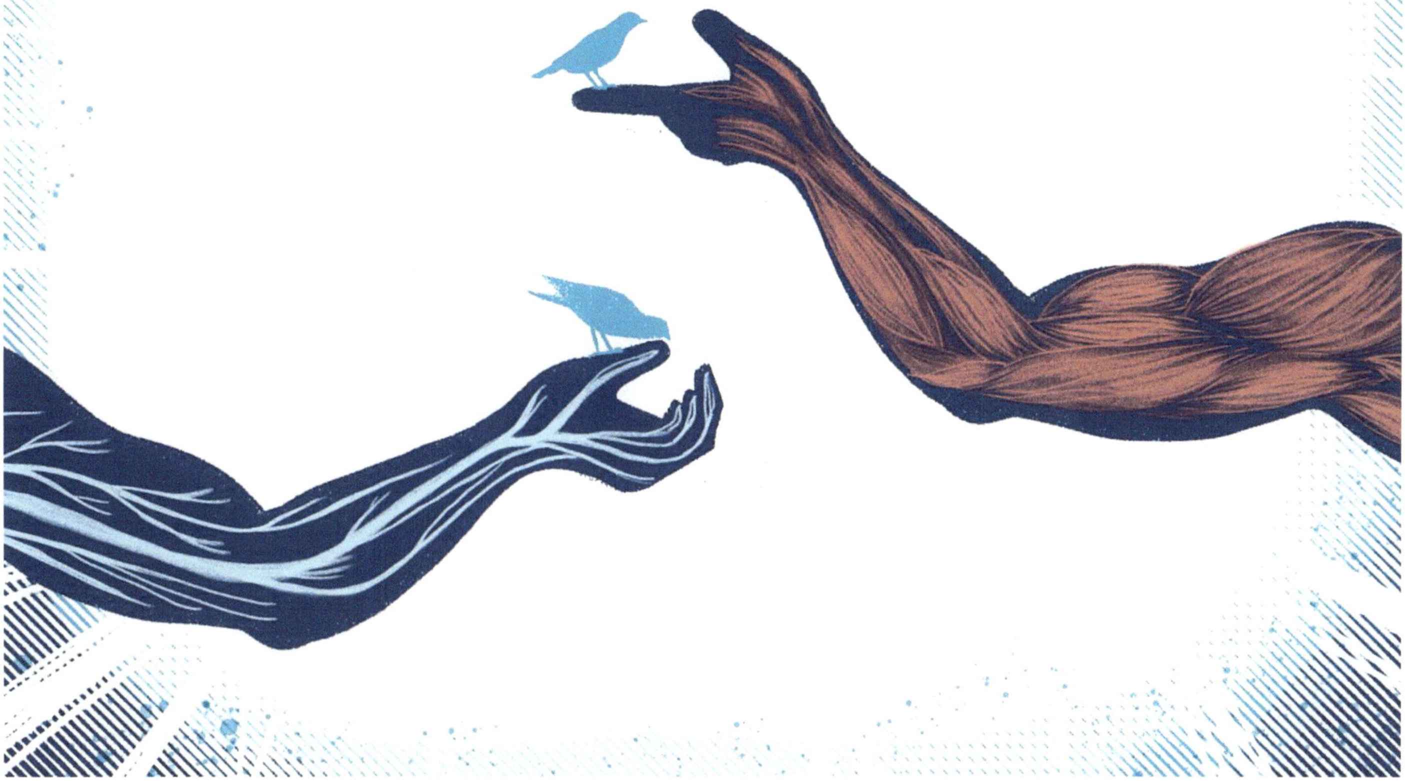

THE ABILITY TO MOVE

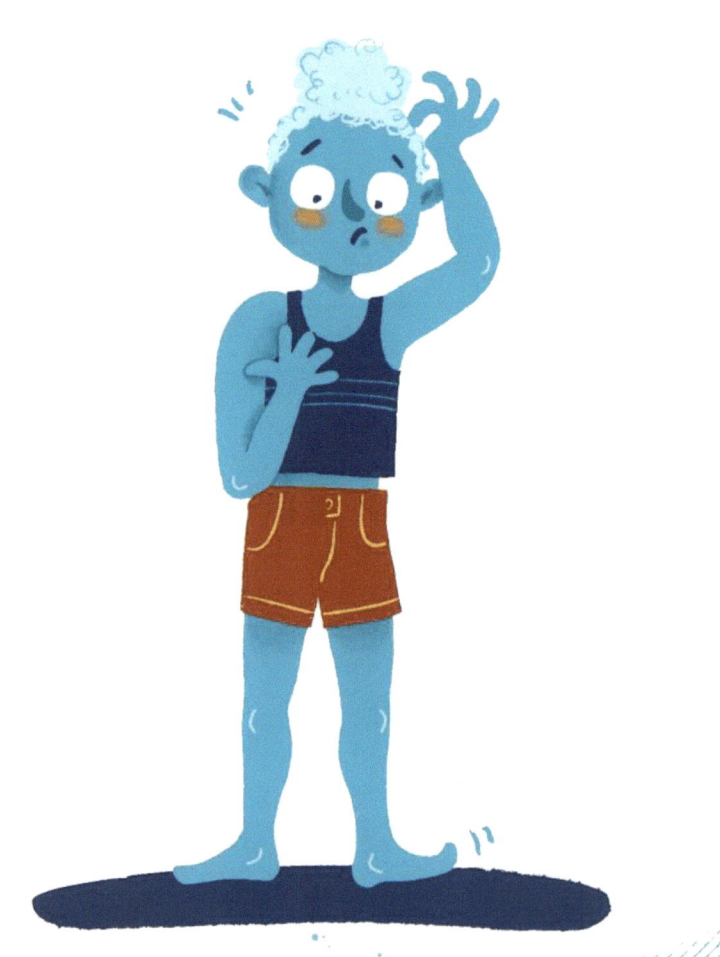

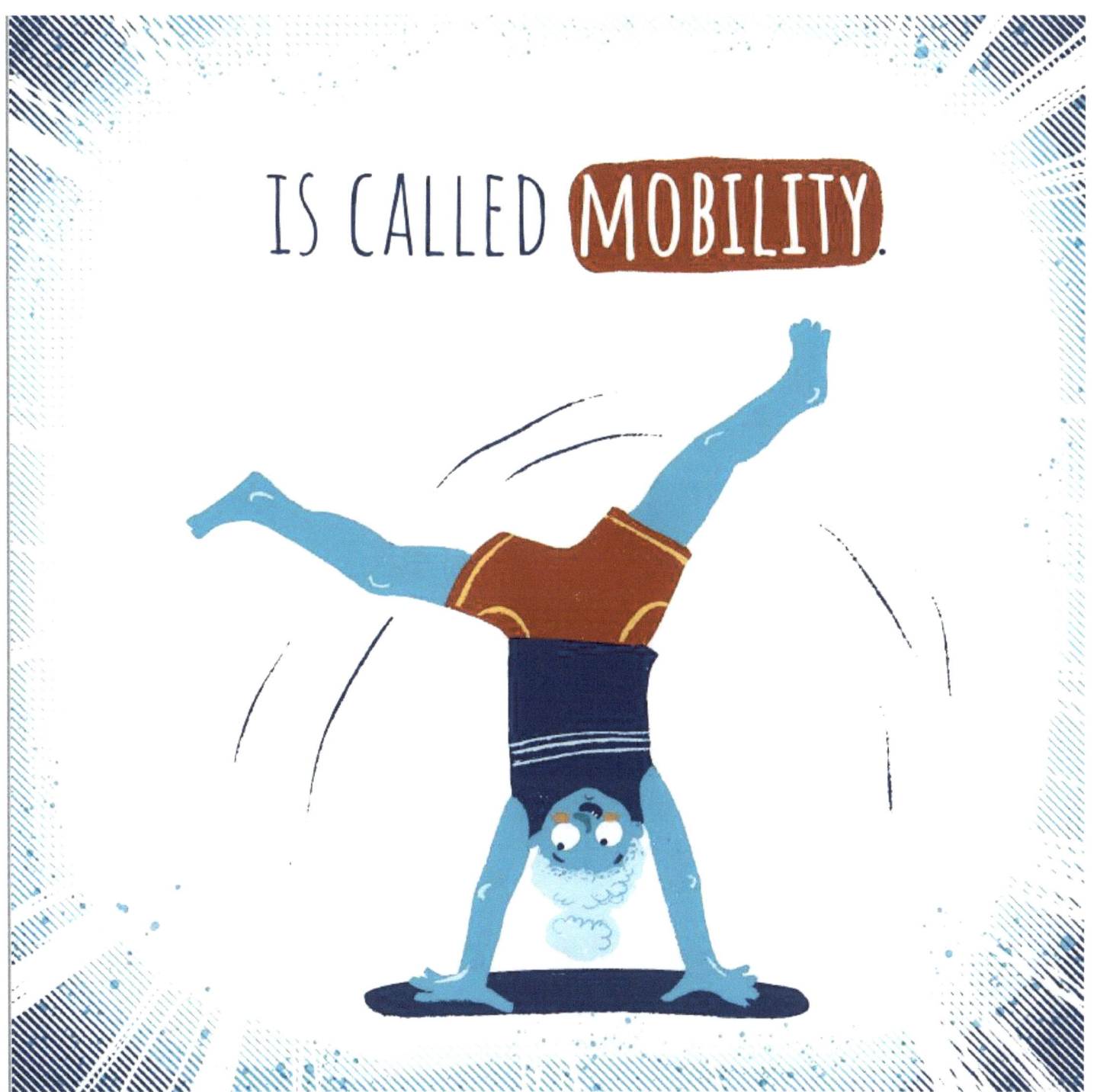

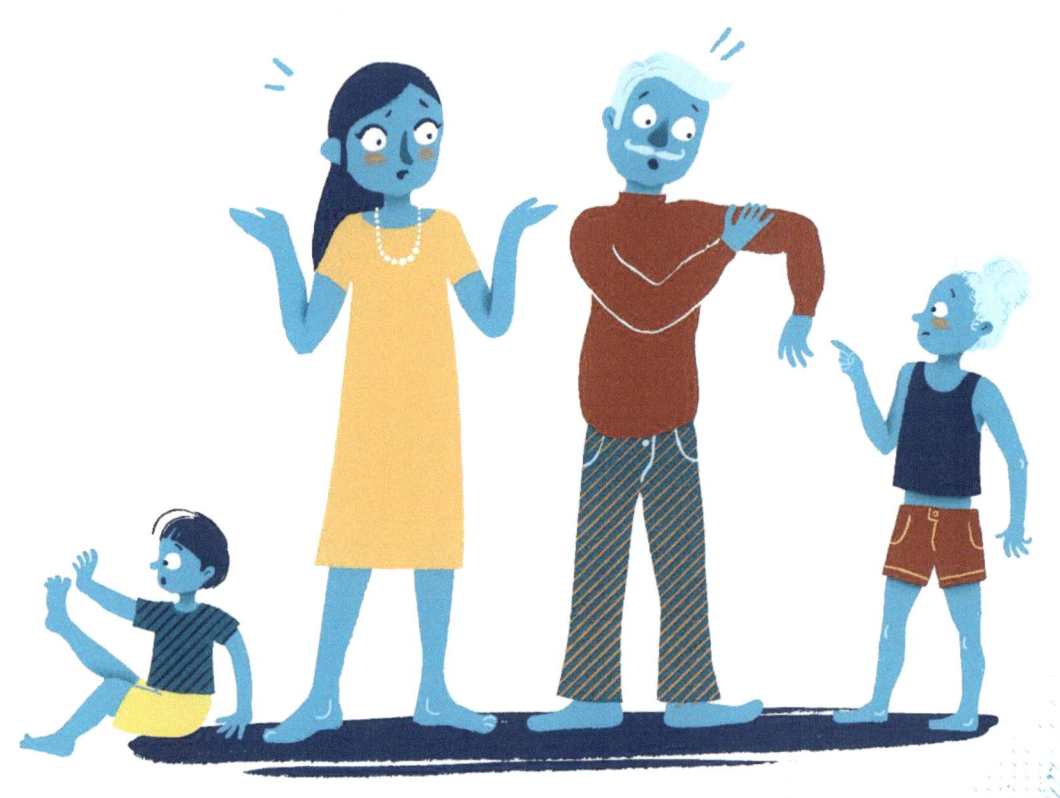

RUN, JUMP, AND PLAY.

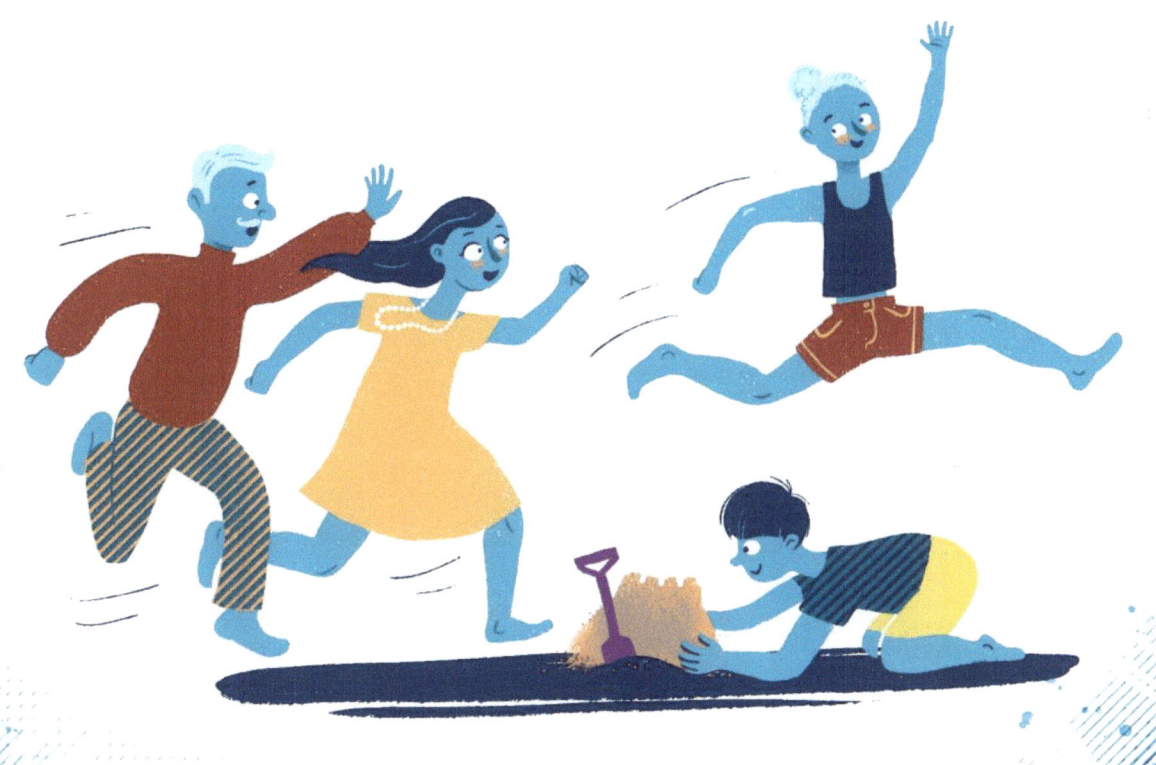

AN INJURY, MEDICAL CONDITION, OR SURGERY

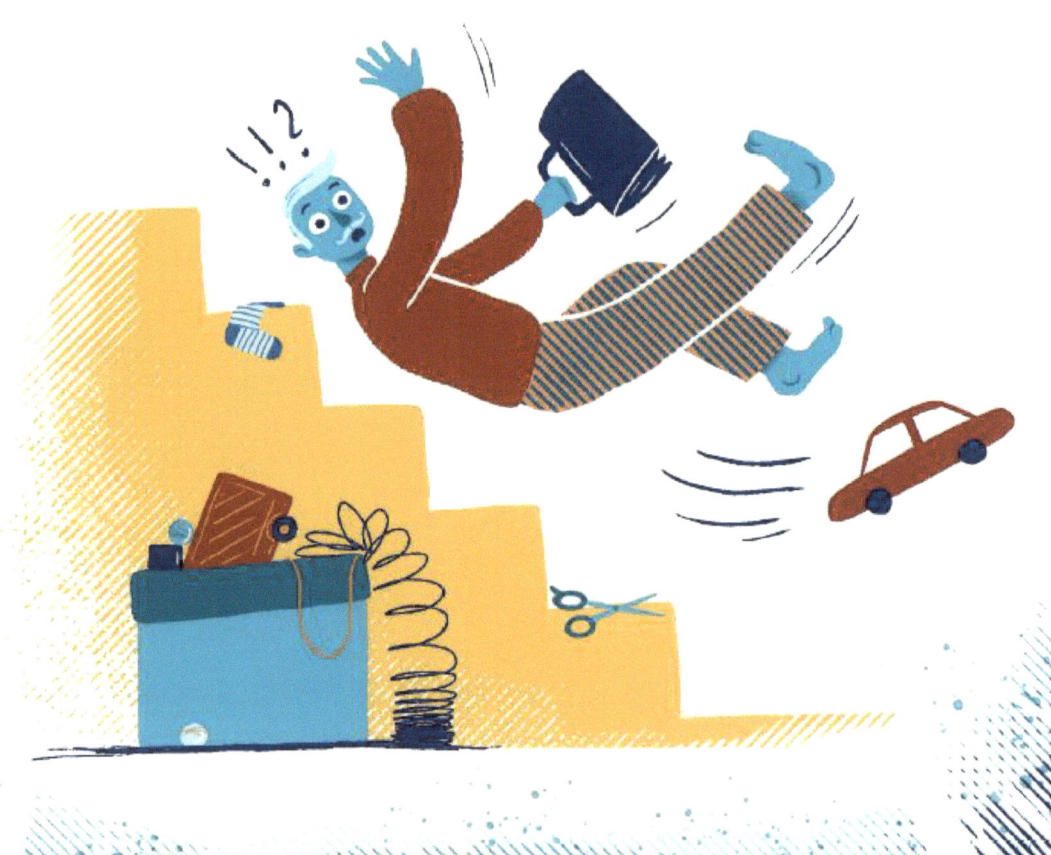

CAN SOMETIMES CAUSE YOUR MOBILITY TO DECREASE.

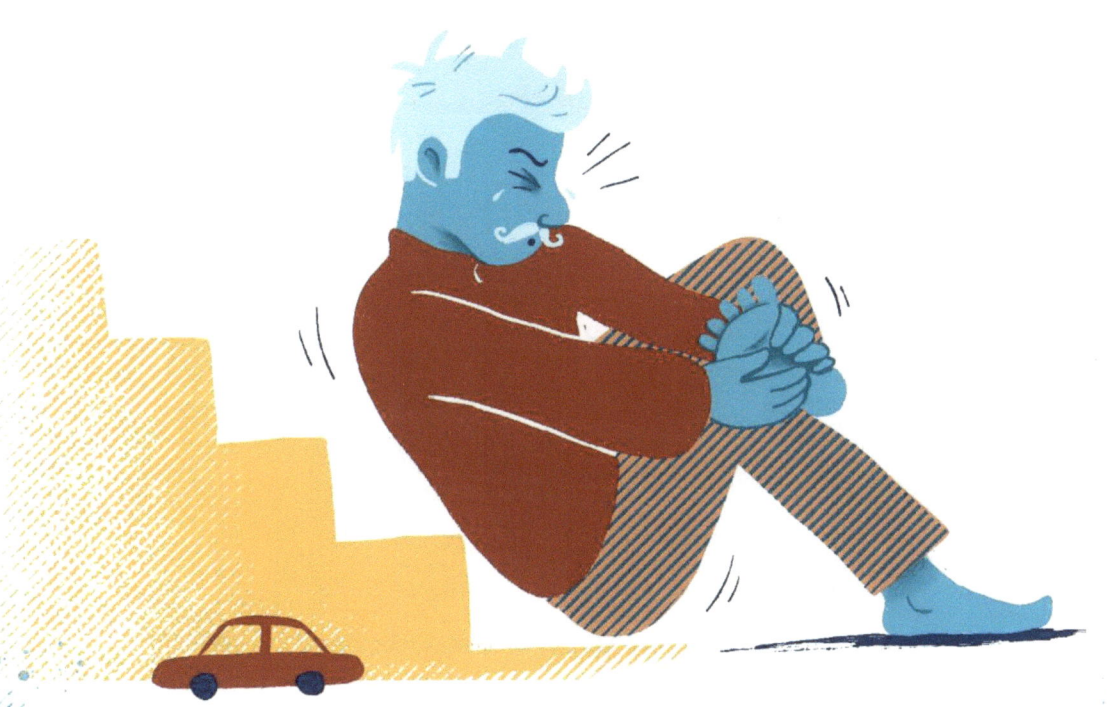

IN ORDER TO RECOVER,

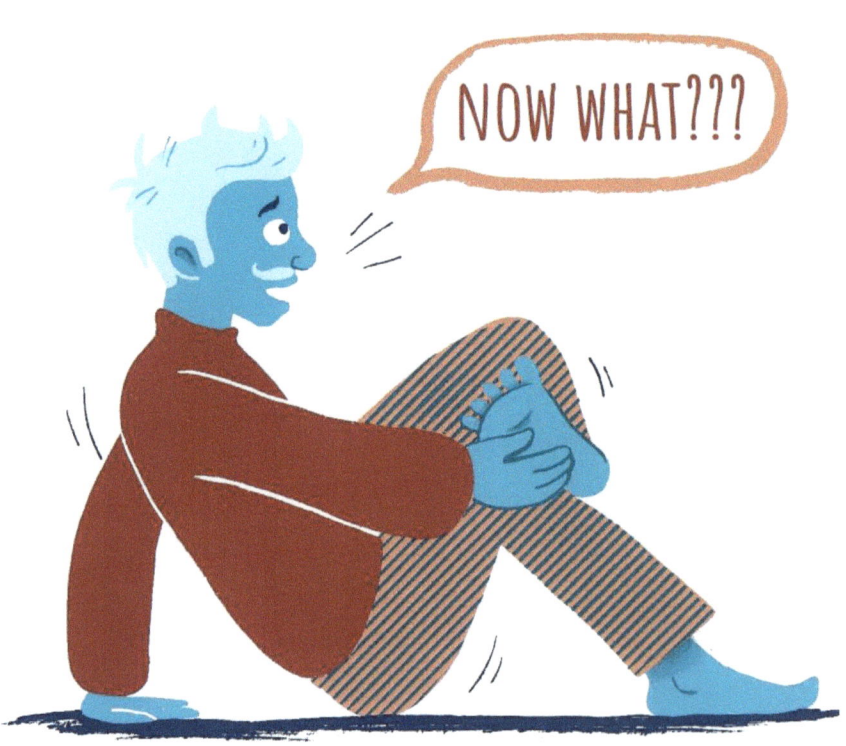

YOU MAY NEED TO VISIT A PHYSICAL THERAPIST.

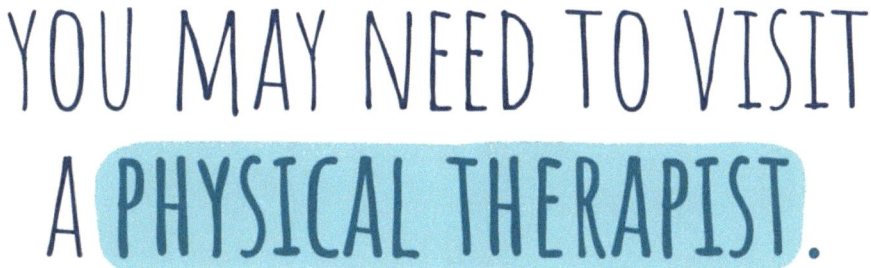

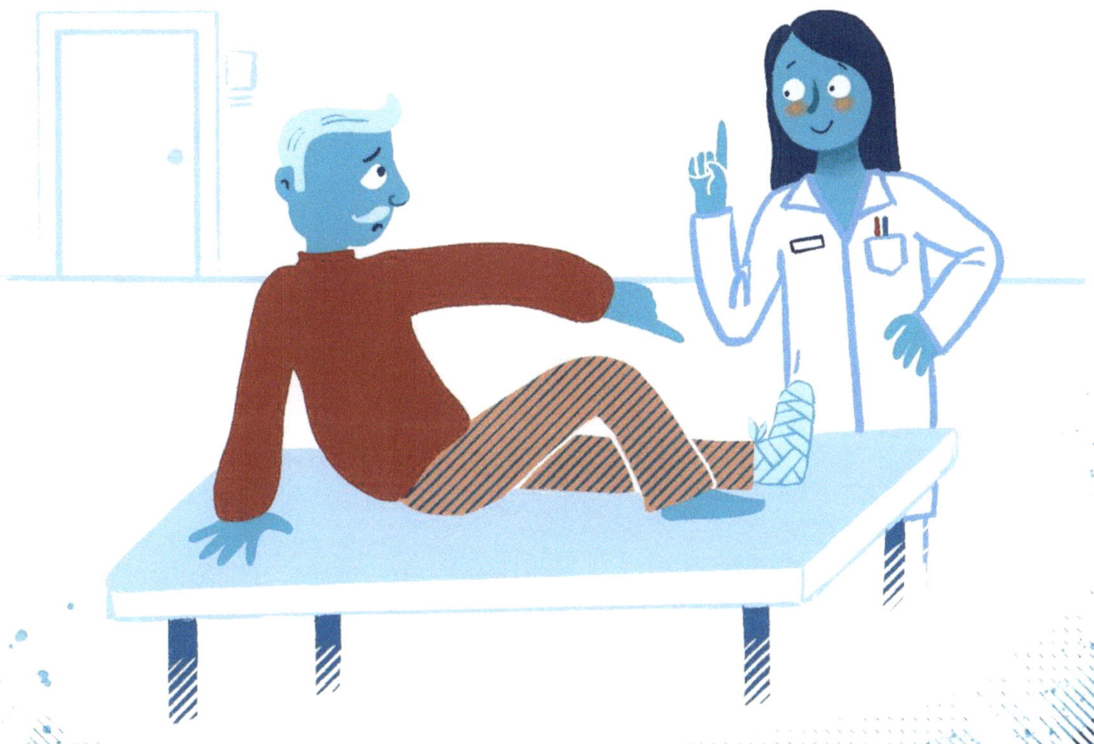

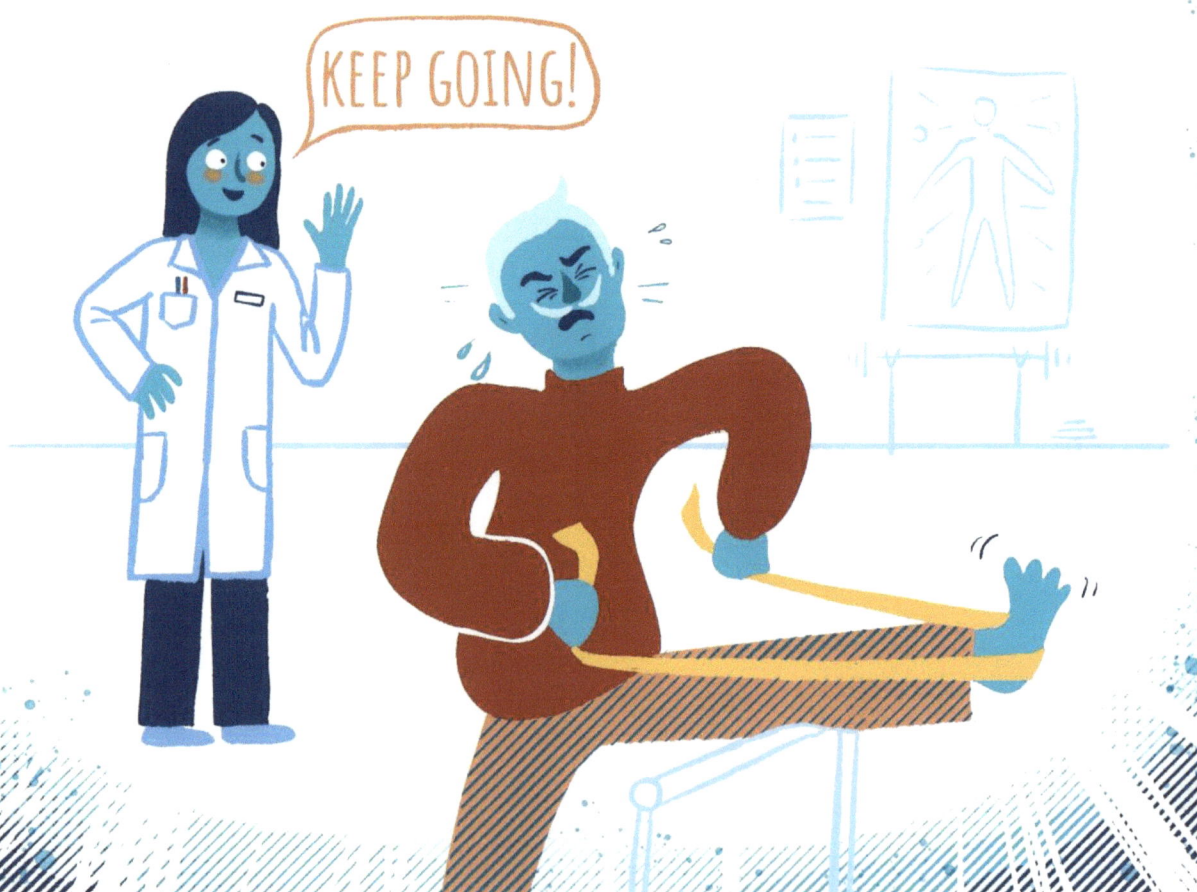

REGAIN YOUR MOBILITY.

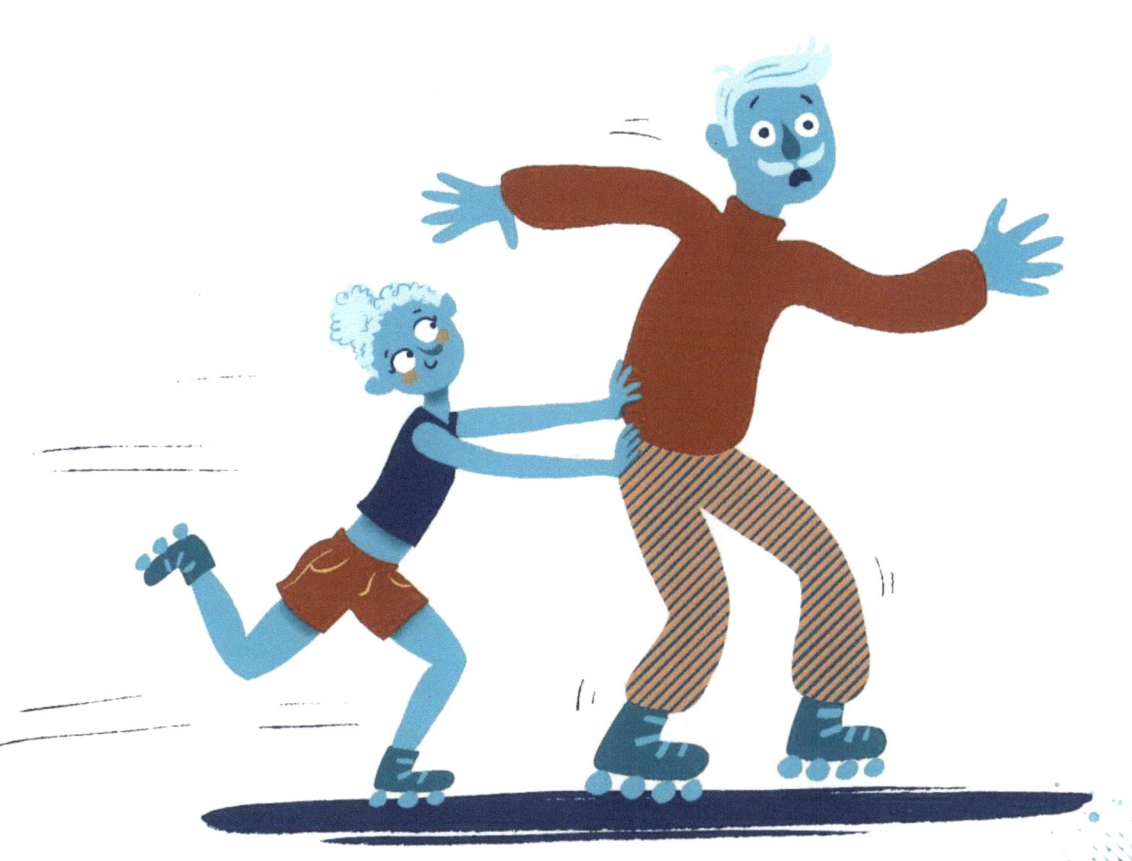

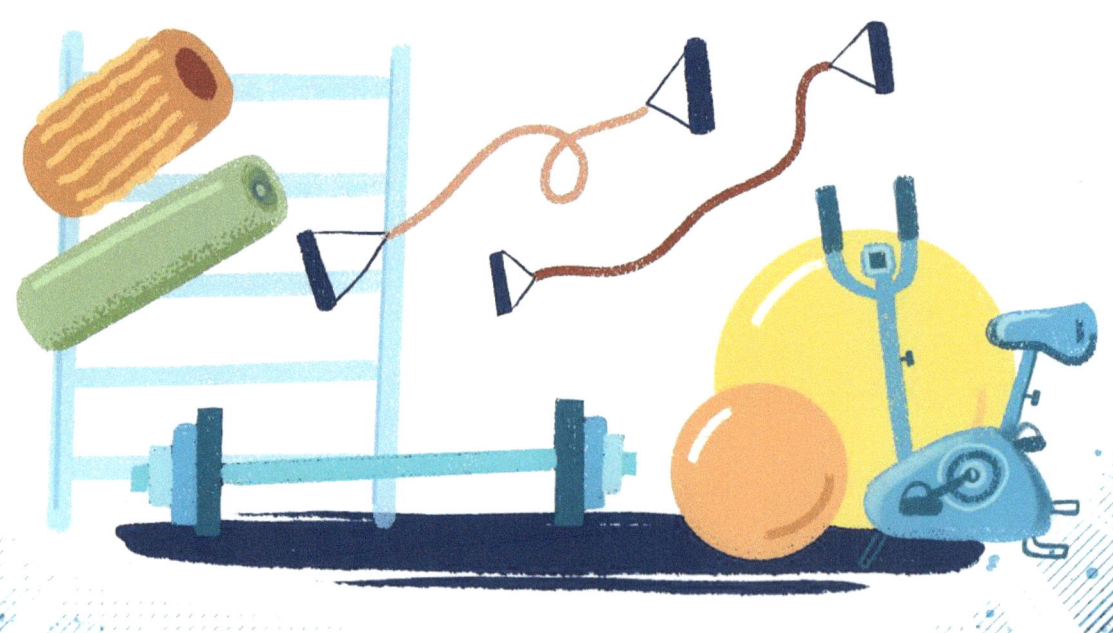

TO IMPROVE STRENGTH AND MOTION.

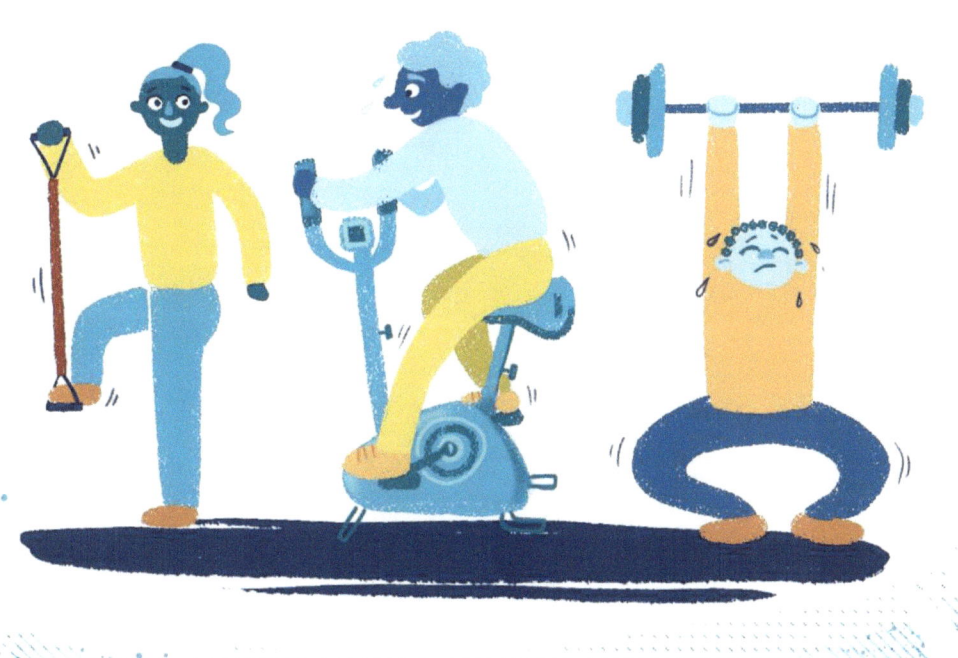

EXCERCISE MEANS MOVING YOUR BODY,

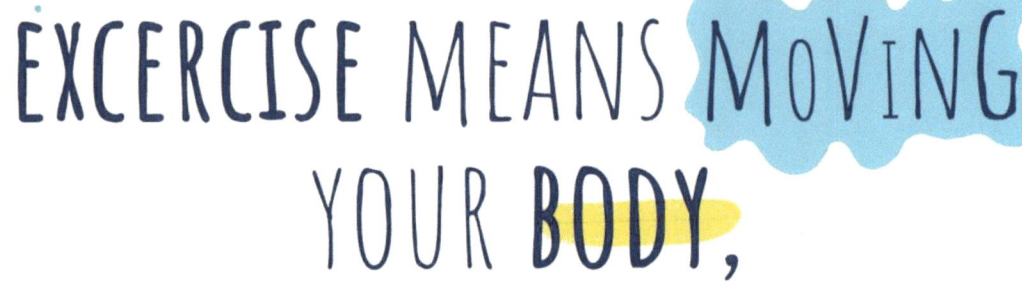

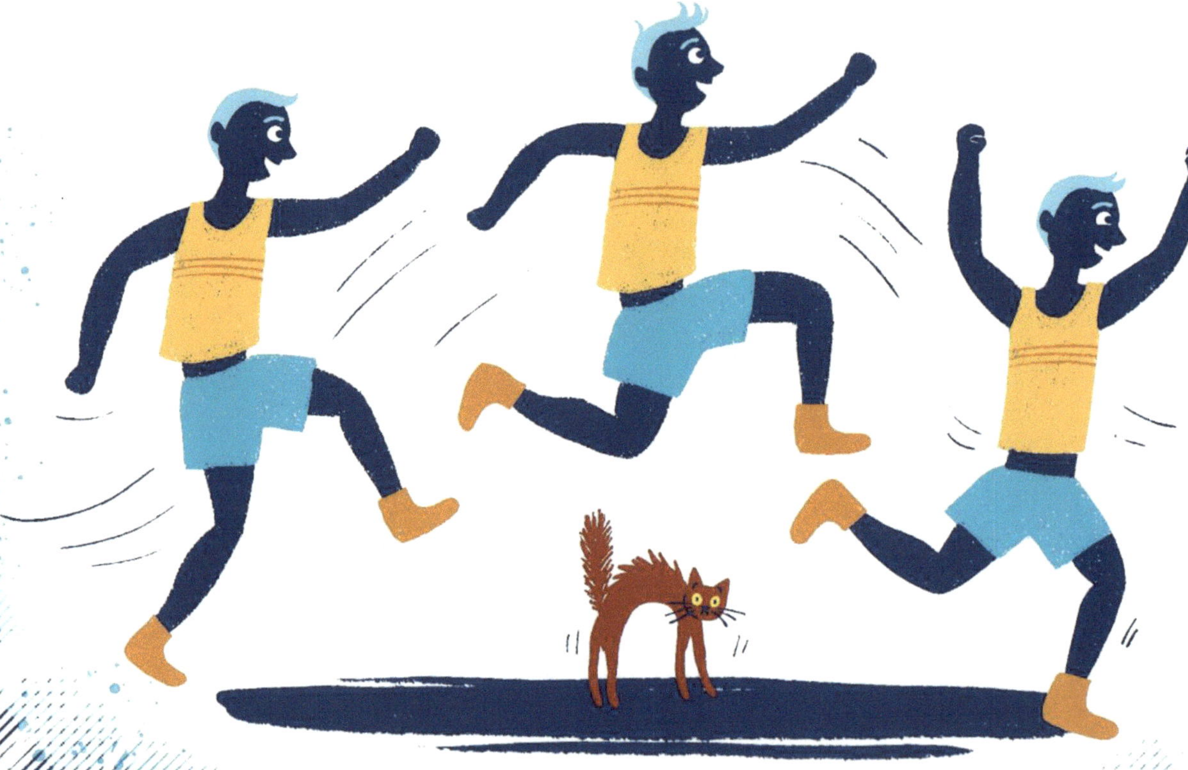

WHICH IS IMPORTANT FOR STAYING HEALTHY!

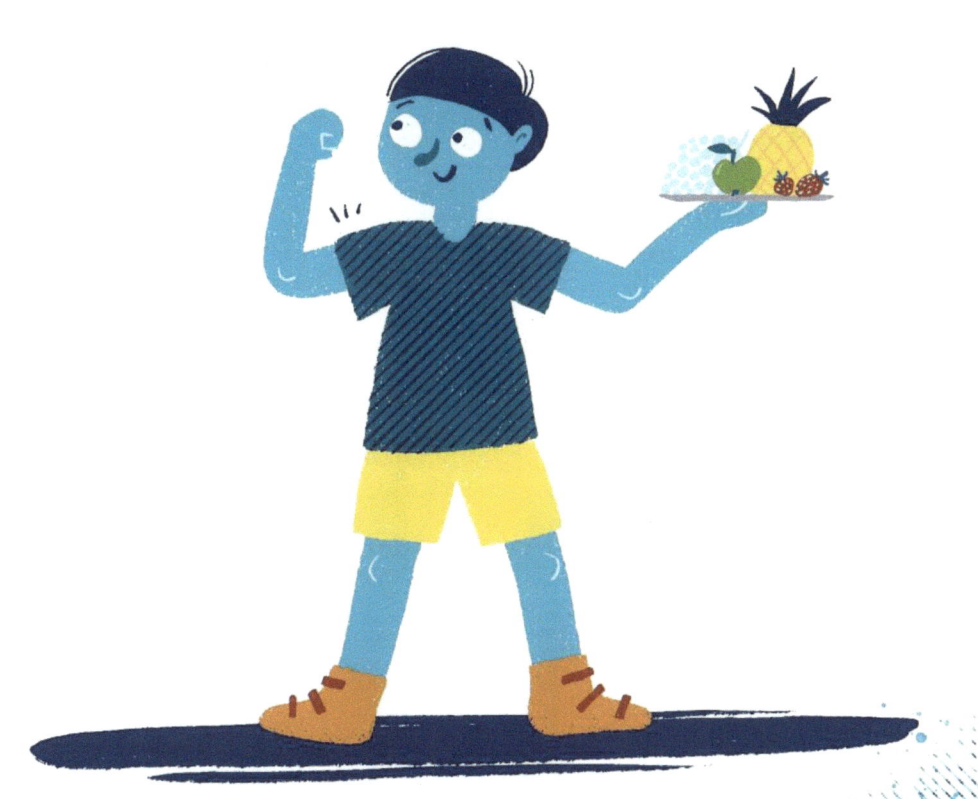

THESE EXERCISES MAY NEED TO BE REPEATED FOR A SHORT

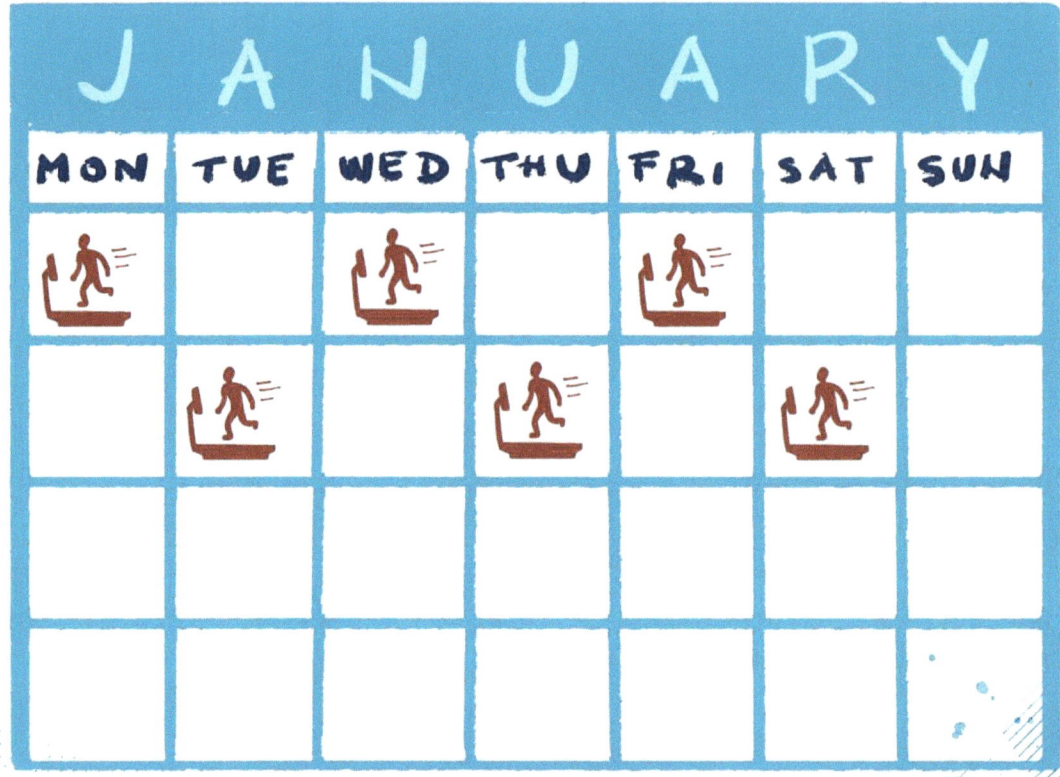

OR **LONG** TIME, DEPENDING ON HOW **BADLY** YOU WERE **HURT**.

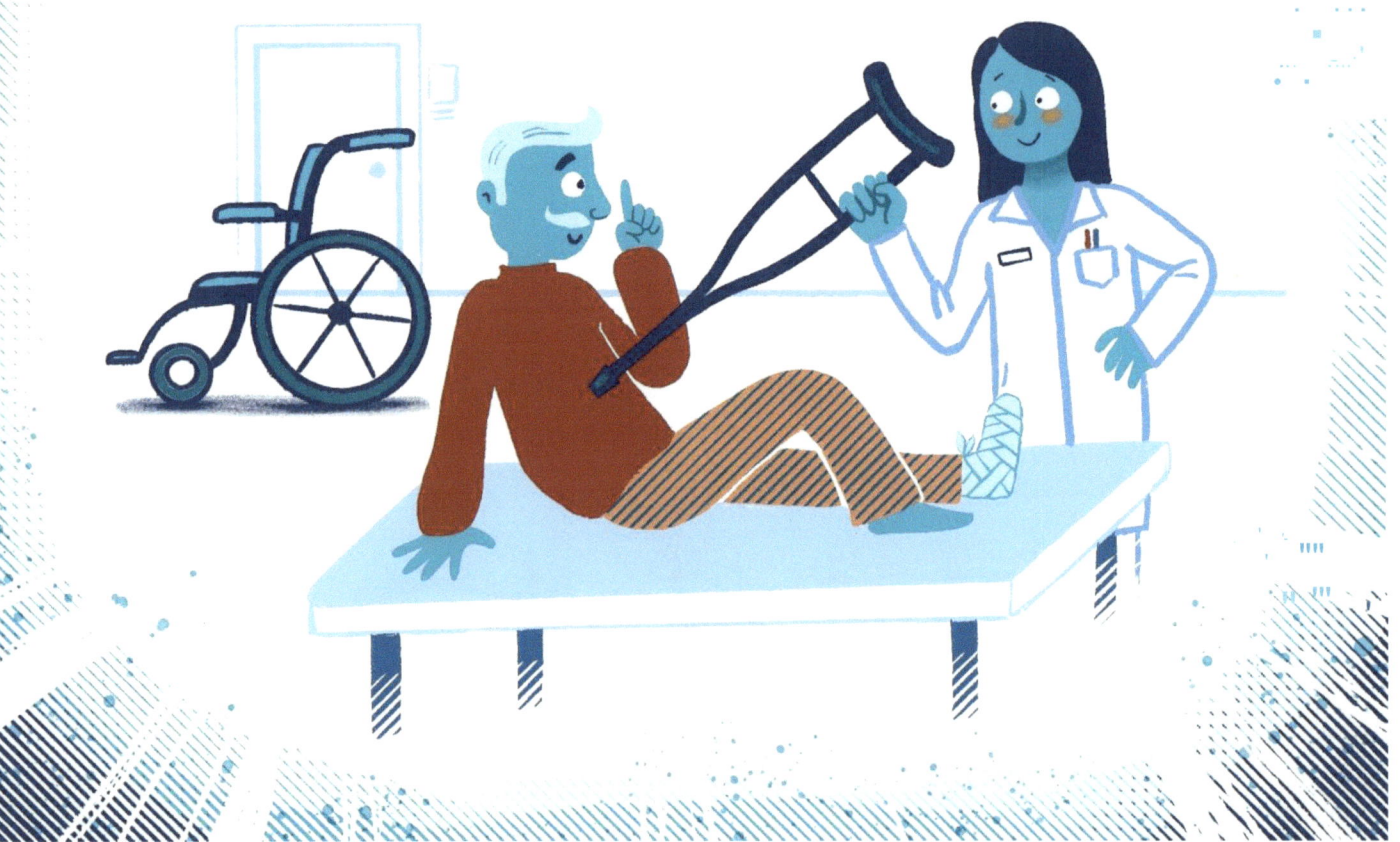

HOW TO USE DEVICES THAT INCREASE THEIR MOBILITY.

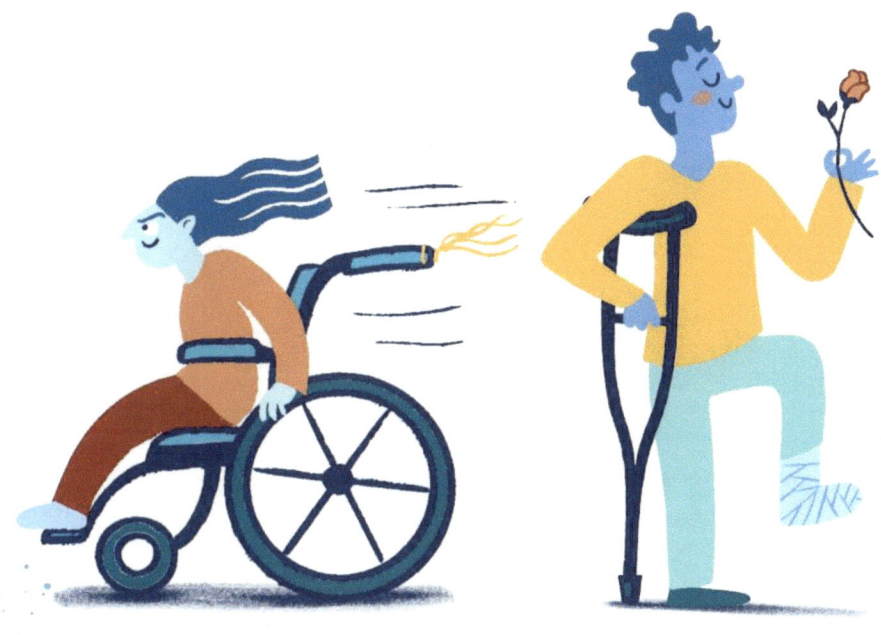

OVER TIME A PHYSICAL THERAPIST CAN HELP YOU

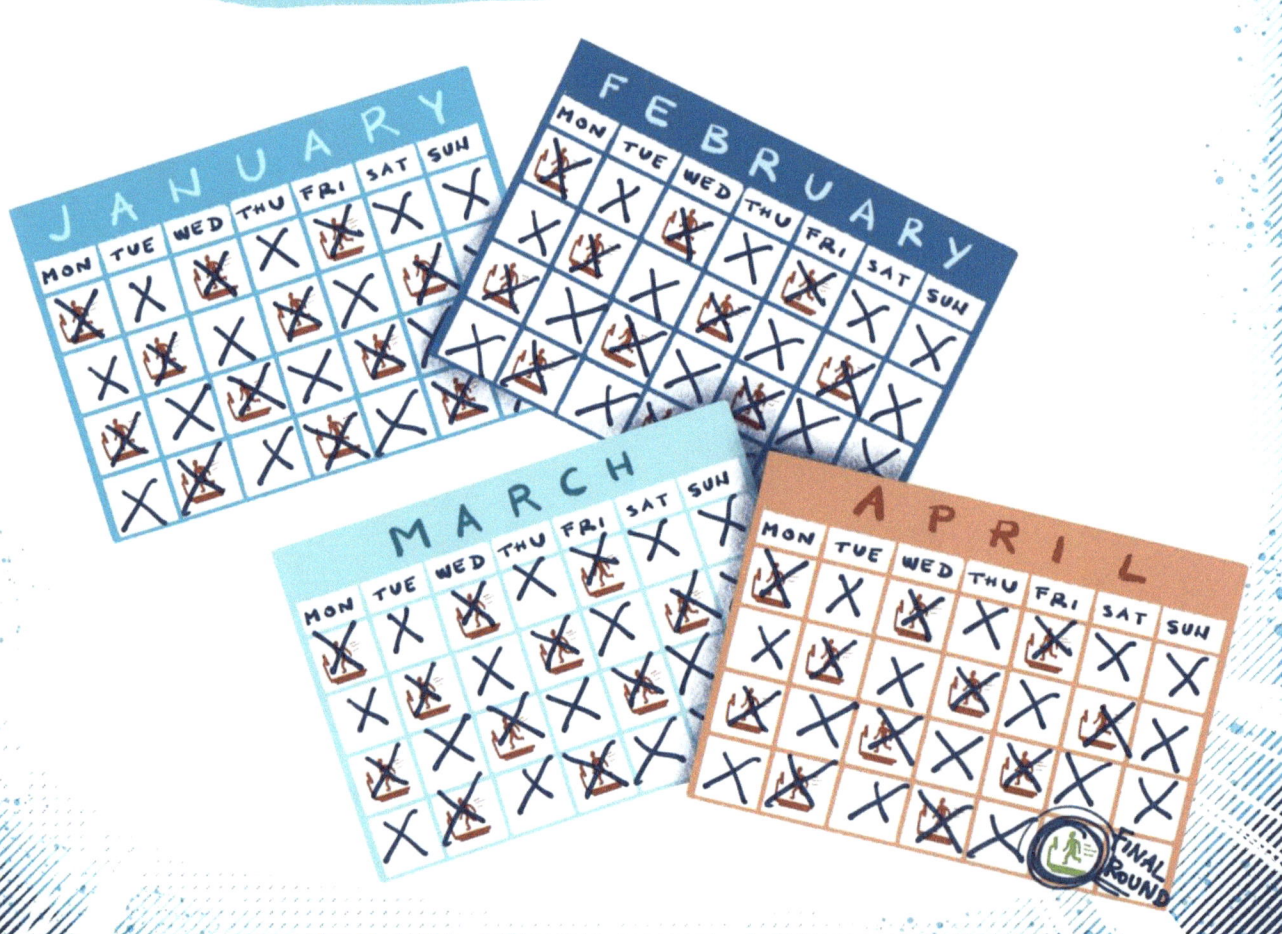

GET **STRONGER** AND DO WHAT'S IMPORTANT TO YOU!

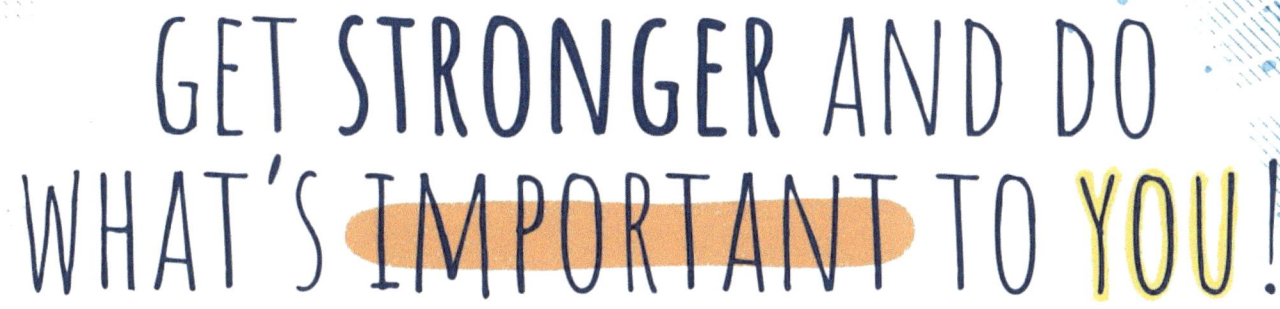

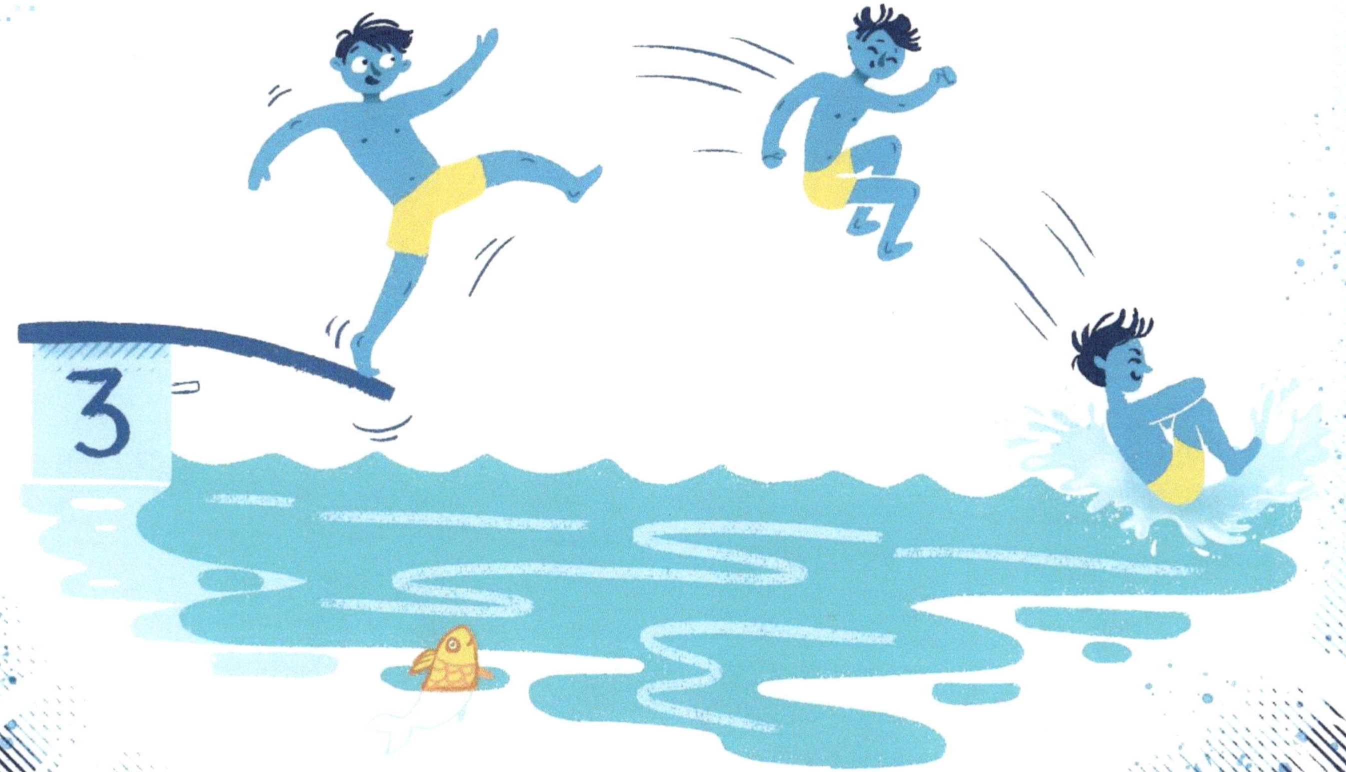

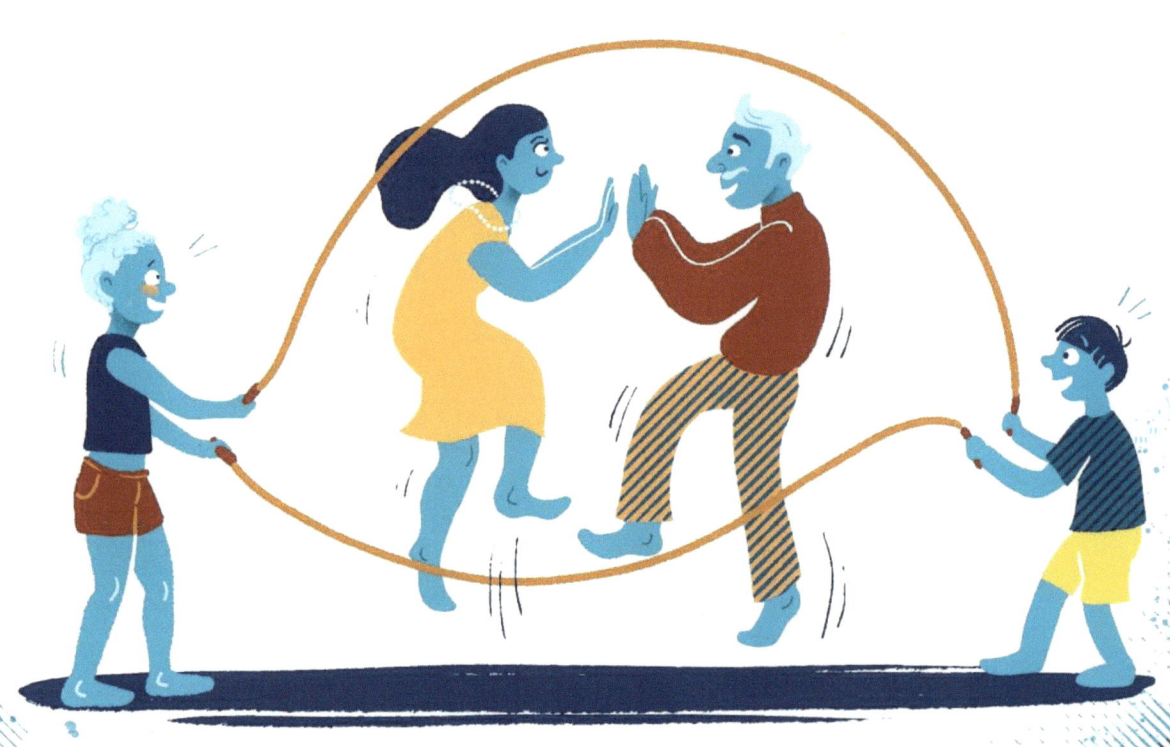

IT'S A GREAT BIG WORLD, WITH LOTS OF OPPORTUNITIES...

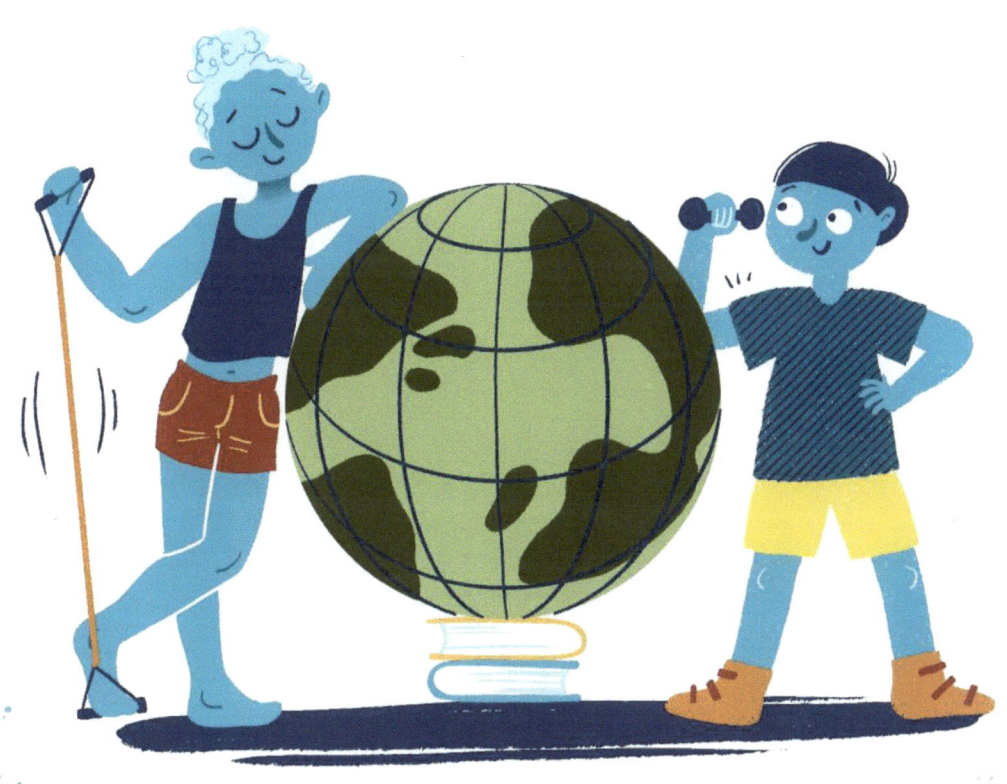

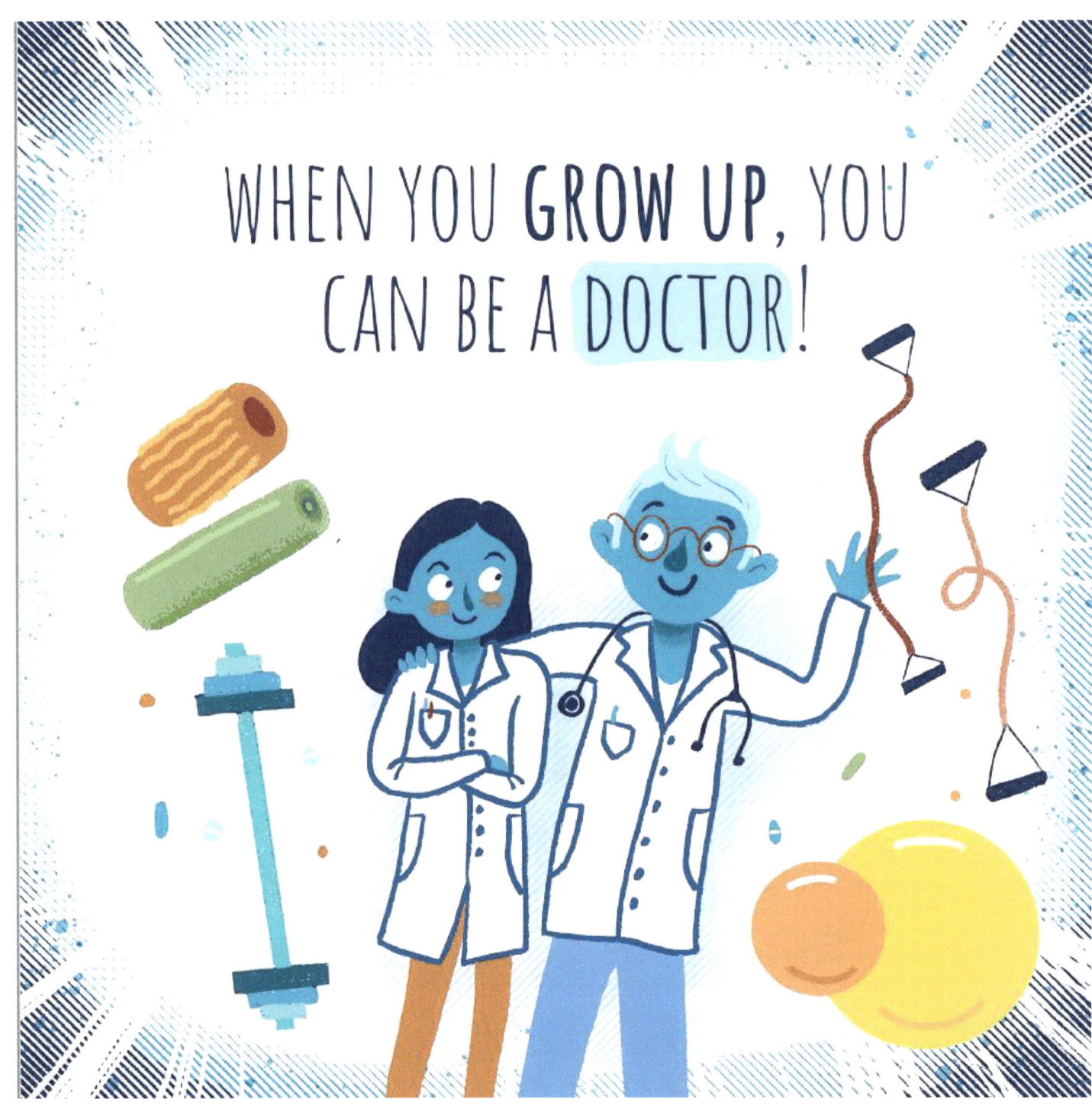

www.ingramcontent.com/pod-product-compliance
Lightning Source LLC
Chambersburg PA
CBHW051832210526
45473CB00005B/1841